Sampiouroman Somé

Evolution of biological tolerance parameters for HIV patients

Evolution of biological tolerance parameters for HIV patients

Sampiouroman Somé

Evolution of biological tolerance parameters for HIV patients

follow-up under arv protocol including DTG in the dermatology and internal medicine departments of CHU-YO

Imprint

Any brand names and product names mentioned in this book are subject to trademark, brand or patent protection and are trademarks or registered trademarks of their respective holders. The use of brand names, product names, common names, trade names, product descriptions etc. even without a particular marking in this work is in no way to be construed to mean that such names may be regarded as unrestricted in respect of trademark and brand protection legislation and could thus be used by anyone.

Cover image: www.ingimage.com

This book is a translation from the original published under ISBN 978-620-6-72025-6.

Publisher:
Sciencia Scripts
is a trademark of
Dodo Books Indian Ocean Ltd. and OmniScriptum S.R.L publishing group

120 High Road, East Finchley, London, N2 9ED, United Kingdom
Str. Armeneasca 28/1, office 1, Chisinau MD-2012, Republic of Moldova, Europe
Printed at: see last page
ISBN: 978-620-8-09527-7

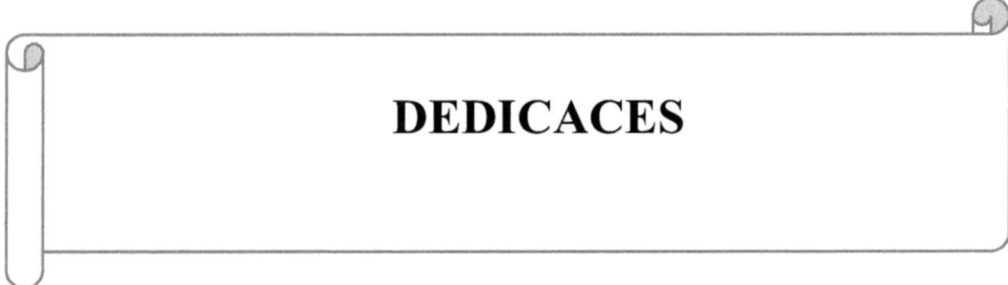
DEDICACES

DEDICACES

To the GOD Father, Son and Holy Spirit

My Lord, you who know hearts; you can read in mine the immense joy, gratitude and need to always walk in your goodness and grace. Everything comes from you Lord, you are my guide and my daily light. I thank you for all the blessings in my life and especially for this wonderful work. Hallowed be thy name.

To my dad SOME Kouakou

Dearest father, no dedication, no words can express the gratitude we feel for you. You instilled in us a sense of fighting spirit, honor and wisdom. You have always been a beacon, the first model and the inspiration of our lives. After so many efforts and sacrifices to give us access to education. We cannot thank you enough, dear father. This work is the fruit of our struggle and we dedicate it to you. May the Almighty give you long life in good health.

To my mother HIEN D. Emeline

Thank you, Mom! Thank you for your prayers, blessings and support. May the Almighty give you long life alongside us, your children.

To my wife Océane K. S. YARO, to you my love, you were always there for me and your advice helped us overcome every obstacle. Thank you for believing in me, for your understanding and patience. This work is yours too. May God keep us together for a long time.

To my son SOME M. Mathis Adrien, fruit of our love, take this work as the most precious object of your life that a father can bequeath to his son. We dedicate it to you as a means of communication whose message you will be able to decode and use to serve your family. May God make you grow in wisdom.

To my big sister Claire Sèohob SOME, family is where life begins and love never ends. Thank you for your infinite love, support and encouragement. Let's stay united. May God strengthen our fraternal ties. Time goes by, everything goes away, but not the love we have for you.

To my aunts and uncles Mwintière SOME, Sansao HIEN, David HIEN, Habraham HIEN, Sambébé SOME, Ingrid HIEN

I am grateful for all your advice, prayers and support. May God bless you and make your activities prosper.

To my cousins,

Thank you for all your advice and encouragement. May God keep us together for a long time.

To my nephews and nieces

Uncle wouldn't have been able to carry out this work without your presence in his life and the smile you send him every time you see him. May the Almighty bless you all and give you the wisdom and intelligence to do better than your parents.

ACKNOWLEDGEMENTS

ACKNOWLEDGEMENTS

Our thanks go to :

To all the teaching staff of the UFR/SDS: it is to your credit that you have accomplished this work, for it is your dedication and self-sacrifice in carrying out your laborious task of transmitting knowledge that have made us what we are. May the quality of your health training, your rigour and excellence in the practice of your profession always be your credo.

To our thesis supervisor: Professor **Estelle YOUL**

Dear Master, in spite of your very precious and busy schedule, you have given importance to this work by guiding us in its realization. For your dedication, promptness and great critical spirit, we thank you most sincerely. May the Lord Almighty bless you and all your family.

To our master and co-director: Dr Désiré SOME

Thank you for your kindness, your constant availability and your kind attention to your students. It arouses in us admiration and unfailing appreciation. From the bottom of our hearts, we thank you. Thank you for the honor you have bestowed on us by making this work possible and by agreeing to supervise it. May God Almighty repay you a hundredfold for the good you have done us.

To our master : Doctor Emile OUEDRAOGO

Dear Master, you accepted without hesitation to co-supervise this work, despite your busy schedule. We admire your scientific rigor, and thank you for your advice and support. May the Almighty watch over you and your family.

To the majors and all the staff of the internal medicine and dermatology departments: your team spirit and family spirit were a great support in the harmonious execution of our work, which was facilitated by the welcome and availability you showed us. Many thanks again.

To my study partners Claver BONKOUNGOU, Lompo TIOYE, Adama SERE

My sincere thanks for the good atmosphere in which we have evolved over the years. May God strengthen this friendship, make it long-lasting and may each of us succeed brilliantly in our socio-professional careers.

To all my friends

As a token of the friendship that unites us and the memories of all the good times we've spent together, I dedicate this work to you and wish you a life full of health, success and happiness.

To the 25ᵉ UJKZ pharmacy graduating class

Happy social and professional careers to all.

TO OUR ESTEEMED MASTERS AND JUDGES

To our honourable Master and Chairman of the jury

Professor Elie KABRE

You are

- ➤ Full Professor of Biochemistry at the UFR/SDS of Joseph KI-ZERBO University;
- ➤ Former Deputy Director of the UFR/SDS at Joseph KI-ZERBO University;
- ➤ Currently Managing Director of the Agence Nationale de Sécurité Alimentaire, de l'Environnement, de l'Alimentation et du Travail (ANSEAT).

Dear master,

We are very grateful for the honor and privilege you have bestowed on us by agreeing to chair the jury for this thesis, despite your busy schedule. We have had the privilege of benefiting from your teaching throughout our university career. Your teaching skills, your extensive medical culture, your approachability and your rigor have always amazed us. May God bless you and shower you and your family with graces.

To our Honorable Master and Thesis Director

Professor Estelle N.H. YOUL

You are

- ➤ Full Professor of Pharmacology at the Unité de Formation et de Recherche en Science de la Santé (UFR/SDS), Joseph KI-ZERBO University;
- ➤ Hospital pharmacist in the hospital pharmacy department at the Yalgado OUEDRAOGO University Hospital;

- Head of Pharmacology, Clinical Pharmacy and Clinical Emergency Toxicology, Department of Hospital Pharmacy, Yalgado OUEDRAOGO University Hospital;
- Deputy Director of the Health Science Training and Research Unit at Joseph KI-ZERBO University.

Dear master,

It is a privilege and an honor to have you as my thesis supervisor. Thank you for entrusting us with this work.

We benefited from your teaching during our training. Your simplicity, your serenity, your scientific rigor, the immensity of your knowledge and your human qualities have always earned our respect.

Dear Master, your hard work and professional dynamism are an example for us to follow.

Please accept, dear master, the expression of our deepest respect and sincere thanks. May God bless you and your family.

To our Honorable Master and Judge

Professor Oumar GUIRA

You are

- Full Professor of Internal Medicine at the Health Sciences Training and Research Unit (UFR/SDS) of Joseph KI-ZERBO University
- Head of Internal Medicine, Centre Hospitalier Universitaire Yalgado OUEDRAOGO (CHU-YO)

We are very grateful for the honor you have bestowed on us by agreeing to judge this work, despite your very busy schedule. We were privileged to benefit from your teachings during our university career, and we remember you as a great man of science, rigorous and committed to a job well done.

May Almighty God grant you a long and happy life. May he continue to bless you and your family.

To our honorable master and co-director

Dr Désiré SOME

You are a pharmacist;

Head of the pharmaceutical dispensing service in the hospital pharmacy department at CHUYO ;

You have agreed to co-supervise this thesis;

We were privileged to benefit from your guidance and advice during our practical training in hospital pharmacy;

We would like to take this opportunity to express our sincere gratitude.

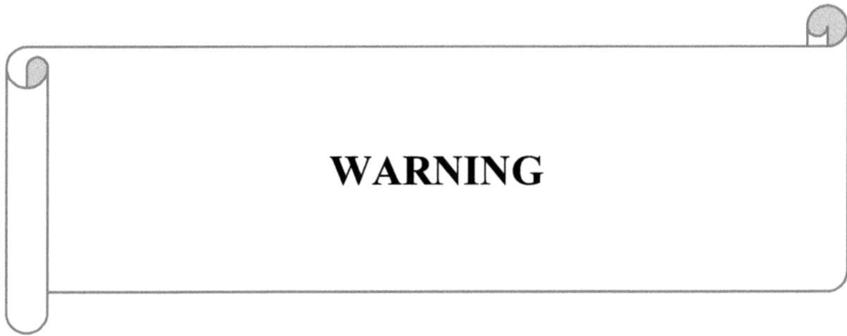
WARNING

TABLE OF CONTENTS

INTRODUCTION/PROBLEM STATEMENT

INTRODUCTION AND PROBLEM STATEMENT

Infection with the Human Immunodeficiency Virus (HIV) constitutes the largest contemporary human pandemic of a constantly lethal infection in the absence of treatment. [13].

HIV infection persists despite efforts to combat it, causing high morbidity and disastrous consequences for families. In addition to prevention, it is important to provide more effective drugs [25].

In 1987, zidovudine was introduced as monotherapy. Triple therapy was introduced between 1995 and 1996, with a combination of protease inhibitors (PIs) and non-nucleoside reverse transcriptase inhibitors (NNRTIs). In 2001, generic drugs were introduced. A decade later, the first preventive treatment known as PrEP (pre-exposure prophylaxis) made its appearance in 2012 [60]. In recent years, WHO-recommended regimens for adults and adolescents have consisted of two types of nucleoside reverse transcriptase inhibitors (NRTIs), accompanied by an NNRTI or PI. Simple regimens, such as fixed-dose combinations and once-daily dosing, are preferred. If necessary, second-line treatment for adults includes two NRTIs combined with a ritonavir-boosted protease inhibitor [56].

Burkina Faso has been combating HIV for over 30 years using a decentralized, participatory approach. HIV prevalence in the general population fell from 7.17% in 1997 to 2.7% in 2003, then to 0.6% [0.6-0.9] in 2022, according to the 2023 report of the United Nations Programme on HIV/AIDS (UNAIDS). [57]. Free treatment in Burkina Faso has been effective at health district level since January 2010 [64]. This has significantly improved ARV coverage, from 31543 in 2010 to nearly 78511 people on ART in 2022 [64]. In the Cadre Stratégique

National (CSN) de lutte contre le sida 2021-2025, the country adopted the "95-95-95" targets for 2025: 95% of people living with HIV (PLHIV) know their HIV status; 95% of PLHIV are on ARV treatment; 95% of patients on treatment have an undetectable viral load [9]. The assessment of the National Multisectoral Plan (PNM) 2022 indicates that the 95-95-95 targets for the fight against AIDS and STIs have been achieved at 89%, 89% and 86% respectively. This assessment is crucial, especially in developing countries [9,38].

In 2019, WHO recommended the priority use of Dolutegravir (DTG) as first- and second-line HIV treatment for all populations, including pregnant women and those of childbearing age, based on evidence. Also, 12 of the 18 countries surveyed by the WHO reported levels of drug resistance exceeding the recommended 10% before treatment with DTG [53]. Dolutegravir is a daily treatment against HIV, with no dietary restrictions. It does not require pharmacological potentiation and offers better protection against HIV resistance. It is well tolerated and effective for both new and treatment-experienced patients. [24]. All the above findings led to the decision to update the 2019 guidelines [53]. Burkina Faso, like other countries, has adopted the new WHO recommendations, advocating the use of DTG [9].

Thus, in the absence of safety data at the national level, the aim of our study is to describe the biological adverse effects of antiretroviral treatments including Dolutegravir in people living with HIV (PLHIV) in order to improve their biological follow-up and management.

PART ONE: GENERAL INFORMATION

I. GENERAL INFORMATION ON HIV INFECTION

1. Epidemiology of HIV infection

1.1 Global situation

According to the UNAIDS in the World 2023 report, 39 million people were living with HIV worldwide at the end of 2022, more than two-thirds of them (25.6 million) in the WHO African Region. However, a 38% decrease in the number of people infected has been observed, from 2.1 million in 2010 to 1.3 million in 2022. In addition, mortality from HIV/AIDS has fallen by 69% since the peak in 2004, and by 51% since 2010, with a global estimate of 630,000 people dying from AIDS-related illnesses in 2022, compared with 1.3 million in 2010. Moreover, this worldwide reduction in lethality is largely due to the availability and accessibility of antiretroviral therapy. Indeed, 29.8 million people had access to antiretroviral therapy in 2022, including 77% of adults over 15 and 53% of children aged 0-14.

Progress in the fight against HIV/AIDS has been significant worldwide, but efforts must continue to reach the "95-95-95" target, which until 2022 was "86-89-93", i.e. 86% of all people living with HIV (PLHIV) knew their serostatus, 89% of them were on life-saving antiretroviral therapy (ART), and 93% of PLHIV on treatment had achieved viral load suppression both to improve their health and to reduce onward transmission of HIV [55].

1.2 The situation in sub-Saharan Africa

Sub-Saharan Africa is the geographic region most affected by the infection, with 25.6 million people, representing 70% of global cases in 2021 [30].

 The UNAIDS 2023 report shows that 4.8 million people in West and Central Africa were living with HIV in 2022. There were 160,000 new infections, including 110,000 new HIV infections among adults aged over 15, and 51,000 among children aged 0-14. The mortality rate is estimated at 120,000 AIDS-related deaths. [58].

In Eastern and Southern Africa, around 20.8 million people will be living with HIV in 2022, with 500,000 cases of new infections, including 450,000 adults over 15 and 58,000 children aged 0-14. The death rate in these regions is around 260,000 AIDS-related cases. [58].

1.3. Situation in Burkina Faso

In Burkina Faso, around 97,000 people, including 16,000 children under the age of 15, were living with HIV in 2020 [21].

HIV prevalence in the general population of Burkina Faso over the past ten years has shown a downward trend. Burkina Faso is classified as a mixed epidemic country, with general population prevalence below 1% and higher prevalence in certain population groups. Indeed, the prevalence of HIV infection in the adult population of Burkina Faso is estimated at 0.6% [10].

This prevalence is quite high in certain population groups, notably sex workers (6.8%); men who have sex with men (MSM) (27.1%); prisoners (2.1%); disabled people (4.6%); drug users (0.5%); healthcare professionals (1.9%) [10].

In relation to the 95-95-95 objective, Burkina Faso recorded the following data on December 31, 2022: 78,511 PLHIV knew their serological status, i.e. a rate of 89%; 78,511 PLHIV were on ARV treatment, i.e. 89%; and 75,511, i.e. 86% of PLHIV on treatment had recorded an undetectable viral load. [9].

2 . HIV/AIDS treatments in Burkina Faso

2.1. Treatment goals and objectives

2.1.1. Purpose of treatment

Combination antiretroviral therapy prevents HIV from multiplying and can clear the virus from the bloodstream. It thus enables the patient's immune system to recover, defeating infections and preventing the development of AIDS and other long-term effects of HIV infection.

2.1.2. Objectives

The overall aim of ART is to improve the quality of life and life expectancy of PLWHA.

Specifically, TARs enable :

- Make the viral load undetectable for as long as possible;
- Lasting restoration of immunity;
- Reduce or eliminate the risk of HIV transmission.

2.2. Classification and mechanisms of action

The different ARV therapeutic classes act at different stages. They are prescribed in the form of multi-drug combinations, often triple therapy, to prevent the virus from becoming resistant to these substances. The different mechanisms of action of ARVs are shown in the figure below. [9] :

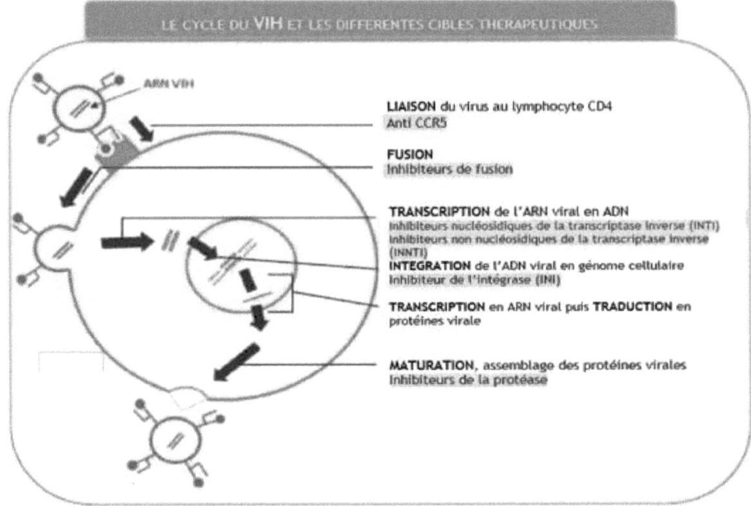

https://vihclic.fr/antiretro-viraux/mode-action-physiopathologie-traitements-antiretroviraux/

Figure 1 ARV action levels [9]

These are [9,34,48] :

❖ Reverse transcriptase inhibitors :

They are subdivided into three subclasses: nucleoside reverse transcriptase inhibitors (NRTIs), nucleotide reverse transcriptase inhibitors (NNRTIs or NNRIs) and non-nucleoside reverse transcriptase inhibitors (NNRTIs or NNRIs). NRTIs block reverse transcriptase by competing with natural nucleosides. NNRTIs block reverse transcriptase by competing with natural nucleotides. NNRTIs act directly by binding to the catalytic site of HIV1 reverse transcriptase; they are inactive on HIV2.

Nucleotides are the organic molecules that make up DNA, RNA and ATP. They are composed of a nucleobase (pyrimidine or purine nitrogen base), a pentose (2'-deoxyribose or ribose) and a phosphate group in the C5' position. When phosphate-free, they are called nucleosides.

- ❖ **Protease inhibitors (PIs)**: prevent the assembly of newly synthesized viral proteins by binding to the protease's catalytic site, thus blocking its proteolytic activity.

- ❖ **Integrase inhibitors (II):** prevent covalent insertion or integration of the HIV genome into the host cell genome by inhibiting integrase catalytic activity.

- ❖ **Fusion inhibitors (FI)**: block fusion between the viral membrane and the target cell membrane, preventing viral RNA from entering the target cell by inhibiting structural rearrangement of HIV1 gp-41.

- ❖ **Capsid inhibitors:** This is a new family of antiretroviral drugs. They work by disrupting the stability of the "shield" that protects the HIV genome and the enzymes it uses to divert CD4 immune cells from creating copies of the virus. This class of antiretroviral drugs has the particularity and advantage over other classes, of being able to intervene at several stages of the replication cycle at once [12].

- ❖ **CCR5 inhibitors:** These are antagonists of HIV membrane co-receptors. They are currently represented by maraviroc (CELSENTRI®). This is a selective and reversible CCR5 [68,72]. Its action is not directed against the virus, but against its target, the CCR5 co-receptor. It prevents the binding of HIV envelope glycoprotein (gp120) to CCR5 coreceptors, thus blocking HIV entry into target cells [2].

- ❖ **N.B.: Pharmacokinetic boosters or potentiators**

A booster is a molecule with the property of increasing the plasma concentration of a drug with which it is associated, notably by inhibiting intestinal and hepatic cytochromes P450. Low-dose ritonavir (100 to 200mg/day) is used for this purpose, not as an antiretroviral. Cobicistat is also used for its booster effect. They have no antiretroviral properties, whatever the dose. [8].

2.3. Pharmacological properties of antiretrovirals

2.3.1. Pharmacokinetic properties of ARVs

The pharmacokinetics of ARVs are summarized in the following table [59,67] :

Table I Summary of pharmacokinetic properties

	F (p. 100)	T_{max} (h)	Fp (p. 100)	Disposal	T1/2 (h)
Abacavir	75 (S)	1	49	kidney + enzymes liver	0,8-1,5
Didanosine	40 (A)	1	< 5	kidney	1-2
Emtricitabine	90 (S)	1	< 5	kidney	9
Lamivudine	80 (S)	1	< 5	kidney	2-3
Zidovudine	60 (S)	1	20	kidney + conjugation	1-1,5
Tenofovir	40 (R)	2-3	< 10	kidney	14
Efavirenz	50 (S)	2-5	99,5	kidney + CYP2B6	50
Nevirapine	90 (S)	4	60	kidney + CYP2B6 + 3A4	25-30
Etravirine	ND	4	99,9	kidney + CYP3A + CYP2C	30-40
Atazanavir	ND (R)	2	86	kidney + CYP3A	7
Darunavir	ND (R)	1-4	94	kidney + CYP3A	10-15
Indinavir	60 (A)	1	60	kidney + CYP3A	1,5-2
Lopinavir /r	ND (R)	5	99	kidney + CYP3A	5-6
Ritonavir	70 (R)	3	99	kidney + CYP3A	3-5
Enfuvirtide	70 (SC channel)	7	97	Peptidases → amino acids	3-8
Maraviroc	25-35 p. 100(S)	2	76	kidney + CYP3A	13

| Raltegravir | ND (R) | 3 | 83 | kidney + UGT1A1 | 9 |

F: bioavailability; T_{max} : time to peak; fp: plasma protein binding; $T_{1/2}$: half-life; S: meal without clinically significant effect; R: meal increases bioavailability, A: fasting (meal decreases bioavailability); ND: not determined.

2.3.2. Therapeutic effects

Available antiretroviral treatments have been shown to reduce the morbidity and mortality associated with human immunodeficiency virus (HIV) infection, but cannot eradicate the virus. [42].

Different classes of antiretroviral drugs work against HIV in different ways, and when combined they are much more effective at controlling the virus and less likely to promote drug resistance than when administered separately. Combination antiretroviral treatments prevent HIV from multiplying and can clear the virus from the bloodstream. It thus enables the patient's immune system to recover, defeat infections and avoid the development of AIDS and other long-term effects of HIV infection [56].

2.3.3. Main adverse effects of antiretroviral treatments

Antiretroviral tritherapies have led to a spectacular reduction in mortality and morbidity linked to HIV infection. However, long-term administration of these drugs leads to undesirable side-effects that can even be life-threatening. Schematically, we distinguish between the toxic effects specific to antiretroviral drugs (mitochondrial toxicity, disorders of glucido-lipid metabolism and hypersensitivity reactions) and the indirect effects of the combination of antiretroviral drugs with other types of medication (cardiovascular accidents linked to metabolic disorders). [22]. The main adverse effects by pharmacological class are as follows:

Table II Summary of adverse effects of ARVs [11]

DCI	Pharmacological classes	Undesirable effects
Zidovudine		Hematological toxicity, Mitochondrial myopathies
Lamivudine	Nucleoside reverse transcriptase inhibitors (NRTIs)	Low-intensity, transient adverse reactions
Abacavir		Hypersensitivity reactions
Emtricitabine		Low-intensity, transient adverse reactions
Tenofovir	Nucleotide reverse transcriptase inhibitor (NRTI)	Hypophosphatemia, Fanconi syndrome (exceptional)
Efavirenz	Non-nucleoside reverse transcriptase inhibitors (NNRTIs)	Rash, Neurosensory disorders
Nevirapine		Cutaneous toxicity, including severe forms (Stevens-Jonhson; Lyell), Hypersensitivity hepatitis
Lopinavir + Ritonavir		Digestive disorders
Atazanavir		Peripheral neurological symptoms, headache, insomnia, vomiting, diarrhea, abdominal pain, nausea, dyspepsia, jaundice, rash, lipodystrophic syndrome, asthenia
Darunavir		Headache, Nausea, Diarrhea
Fosamprenavir		Nausea, hypertriglyceridemia, hypercholesterolemia, hyperglycemia
Raltegravir	Integrase inhibitor (II)	Vertigo, arthralgia, asthenia, abdominal pain, pruritus, hepatic cytolysis
Dolutegravir		Diarrhea, headaches, insomnia, nausea, dizziness, hypersensitivity rash, severe liver damage

| Enfuvirtide | Fusion inhibitor (FI) | At the injection site: redness, pain, small balls. |
| Maraviroc | Input inhibitor | Cough, fever, lung infection, rash, muscle and abdominal pain, dizziness, constipation, itching, difficulty sleeping |

2.4. Antiretroviral treatments available in Burkina Faso

Table III Main antiretroviral molecules by pharmacological group [9]

Molecules	Adult dosage
Nucleoside reverse transcriptase inhibitors (NRTIs)	
Abacavir (ABC)	300mg twice a day or 600mg once a day
Emtricitabine (FTC)	200mg once a day
Lamivudine (3TC)	150mg twice a day or 300mg once a day
Zidovudine (AZT)	200-300mg twice a day
Nucleotide reverse transcriptase inhibitors (NRTIs)	
Tenofovir (TDF)	300mg once a day
Tenofovir alafenamide (TAF)	25 mg once a day
Non-nucleoside reverse transcriptase inhibitors (NNRTIs)	
Efavirenz (EFV)	600 mg once daily or 400 mg once a day
Nevirapine (NVP)	200 mg once a day for 14 days, then 200 mg twice a day
Etravirine(ETV)	200 mg twice daily
Rilpivirine*(RPV)	25 mg once a day
Protease inhibitors (PIs)	

Lopinavir/ritonavir (LPV/r)	400 mg/100mg twice daily
Darunavir (DRV)	800 mg+100 mg ritonavir once daily or 600 mg+100mg ritonavir twice daily
Atazanavir/ritonavir (ATV/r)	300 mg/100mg once a day

Table IV Main antiretroviral molecules by pharmacological group (Continued)

Molecules	Adult dosage
Ritonavir (RTV)	Dosage according to combination
Fosamprenavir/ritonavir (FPV/r)	700 mg+100 mg twice daily
Integrase (II) inhibitors	
Raltegravir (RAL)	400mg twice daily
Dolutegravir (DTG)	50mg once daily (twice daily in non-II-naive patients)
Fusion inhibitors (FI)	
Enfuvirtide * (T20)	90mg twice daily subcutaneous injection
CCR5 antagonists	
Maraviroc (MVC)	150 to 600 mg twice a day

*Molecules marked with an asterisk are not available in Burkina Faso.

❖ **Preventive ARV treatment or pre-exposure prophylaxis (PrEP)**

Pre-exposure prophylaxis (PrEP) is a drug-based prevention method using the following molecules:

-Tenofovir (TDF) monotherapy or ;

-A fixed combination of Tenofovir/Emtricitabine or Lamivudine or ;

Sustained-release injectables such as Cabotegravir or ;

Extended-release vaginal rings, such as the vaginal ring containing Dapivirine.

These treatments are used as a preventive measure, enabling HIV-negative people to avoid infection even if they come into contact with the virus. As the name suggests, it is used "prior to exposure" to HIV. It is also indicated for people at "substantial risk", defined as a risk of contracting HIV greater than 3 per 100 person-years. [9].

❖ Injection treatments

Since December 21, 2021, injectable treatments marketed by ViiV Healthcare have been available for the treatment of HIV infection. This is a new combination of an integrase inhibitor and a non-nucleoside reverse transcriptase inhibitor, namely cabotegravir and rilpivirine respectively, injectable every two months with a prolonged action profile. [1].

❖ Chemoprophylaxis

Chemoprophylaxis is not antiretroviral treatment, but a strategy aimed at using drugs in PLWHIV to reduce the onset of opportunistic infections (primary prophylaxis) or the recurrence of a previously treated and cured infection (secondary prophylaxis).

Primary prophylaxis mainly uses cotrimoxazole, while secondary prophylaxis uses cotimoxazole, acyclovir, fluconazole or the combination of pyrimethamine+clindamycin+folinic acid or pyrimethamine+sulfadiazine+folinic acid [11].

2.5. Therapeutic protocols in Burkina Faso

The recommended combination therapy is three (3) ARVs or triple therapy with two different ARV classes:

2 IN + 1 II" combination: indicated in cases of HIV1 or HIV2 infection, or HIV-1 and 2 co-infection. [50].

Table V Choice of first-line molecules for HIV1, HIV2 and HIV1+2

First-line ARV	Schematics
Recommended layout	TDF/FTC or 3TC / DTG
Alternative schemes	TDF/FTC or 3TC/EFV 400 AZT /3TC + EFV 600 AZT/3TC+DTG TDF/3TC or FTC + LPV/r

NB: In the case of HIV-2, it is imperative to use regimens containing DTG or LPV/r. An ABC-based regimen may be used in cases of renal failure.
 Alternative regimens will be used in the event of contraindication or toxicity to one or more molecules in the preferred first-line regimen. The offending molecule will be replaced as follows, taking into account the severity of the side effect.
A first-line regimen is considered to be any first-line regimen in an antiretroviral treatment-naive subject. Any substitution in the event of intolerance, for example, is also considered a first-line regimen. [22].

Table VI Second-line ARV protocols in Burkina Faso

HIV type	First-line treatment	Recommended second-line treatment	Alternative second-line treatment

HIV1	TDF/FTC or 3TC/DTG	AZT / 3TC+ ATV/r	AZT/3TC+LPV/r
	TAF/FTC or 3TC +. DTG	ABC / 3TC+ ATV/r	ABC/3TC + LPV/r
	TDF /FTC or 3TC/ EFV	AZT / 3TC+ DTG	ABC / 3TC+ ATV/r or LPV/r
	AZT/3TC+EFV	ABC / 3TC+ DTG	AZT / 3TC+ ATV/r or LPV/r
		TDF/3TC/DTG	TDF/FTC+DTG
		ABC/3TC+DTG	TDF/FTC+ ATV/r or LPV/r
			ABC/3TC+ ATV/r or LPV/r
HIV2 and HIV1 &2	TDF/FTC or 3TC/DTG	AZT/3TC+ LPV/r	AZT/3TC+ DRV/r
	TAF/FTC or 3TC +. DTG	ABC/3TC+ LPV/r	ABC/3TC + DRV/r
	TDF/FTC+ LPV/r	AZT/3TC+DTG	ABC/3TC+DRV/r
		ABC/3TC+DTG	AZT/3TC+ DRV/r
	AZT/3TC + LPV/r	TDF/3TC/DTG	TDF/FTC+DTG
		ABC/3TC+DTG	TDF/FTC or 3TC + DRV/r
			ABC/3TC+DRV/r

2.6. Current recommendations in Burkina Faso

Table VII Recommended first-line regimen for adults, including pregnant women and adolescents weighing over 35 kg

Populatio n category	1st line option recommended	Alternatives for the 1st line
Adults, adolescents over 35 kg and pregnant women	TDF/3TC/DTG	TDF/3TC (OR FTC)/EFV (400mg) AZT/3TC+DTG AZT/3TC+EFV (400mg)

New PLHIV are systematically enrolled in the TLD unless contraindicated. [43].

Since 2019, Dolutegravir and low-dose Efavirenz in combination with two NRTIs can be used for first- or second-line treatment, and Darunavir/ritonavir remains the anchor drug for third-line treatment. The use of dual therapies combining Dolutegravir and Lamivudine, for initial treatment, is also possible under certain conditions [54].

The first-line strategy remains that of combining several molecules from different classes. First-line treatment classically comprises 2 NRTIs and a 3ème agent from a different class. This 3ème agent has evolved over time: PI boosted by Cobicistat or Ritonavir, NNRTIs and, more recently, integrase inhibitors [33].

2.7. The case of Dolutegravir

On the basis of new evidence on benefits and risks, the World Health Organization recommends the preferential use of Dolutegravir (DTG) as a first- and second-line HIV treatment for all populations, including pregnant women and those of childbearing age [53].

An effective substance with few side effects, DTG is one of the most widely used antiretrovirals today (27% of third agents used; 2018 data from Toulouse University Hospital). A relatively recent antiretroviral (marketed in France since 2014), it has shown its value in the combined form with two NRTIs in triple therapy. DTG is also useful in dual-therapy tapering strategies with Rilpivirine, and potentially with a nucleoside inhibitor such as Lamivudine. On the other hand, DTG has shown no benefit as a monotherapy strategy. Indeed, virological failures, with selection of resistance mutations, have been frequently observed.

2.7.1. Dolutegravir mechanism of action

The integrase inhibitor class represents the most recent antiretroviral family to be developed and made available as part of therapeutic strategies. After fusion of the virion with the membrane, viral RNA is released and retro-transcribed into double-stranded DNA, a step specifically targeted by nucleos(t)idic and non-nucleosidic reverse transcriptase inhibitors. This DNA is then transported to the cell nucleus, where it integrates into the host cell's genome. This is the precise stage targeted by integrase inhibitors.

2.7.2. Pharmacological properties of DTG
❖ Pharmacokinetics
The pharmacokinetics of DTG were linear over a dose range from 10 to 50 mg. DTG has a half-life of 24h (T1/2=24h) [62].
DTG absorption is rapid (Tmax = 2.5 h). DTG absorption and exposure are affected by meal intake and composition.
DTG is highly bound to plasma proteins (>99%). Albumin is the main transport protein for DTG in the vascular compartment. Alpha-1-acid glycoprotein is involved to a lesser extent in DTG binding in the blood.

Uridine diphosphate (UDP)-glucuronosyltransferase (UGT) 1A1 is the main enzyme involved in DTG metabolism. Other minor pathways include cytochrome P450 3A4 (CYP450) and UGT1A3 and 1A9. DTG has no inhibitory or inductive action on these three enzymes or on other CYPs (1A2, 2A6, 2B6, 2C9, 2C19, 2D6, 2B7). The metabolites have no antiretroviral activity of interest.

DTG is eliminated mainly in the faeces (64%), in the form of parent substance and metabolites. DTG is also excreted in the urine (31.6%), mainly as a glucuroconjugate metabolite, resulting from metabolism by UGT1A1. Metabolites resulting from oxidation reactions (CYP3A4 pathway) are also eliminated renally [47].

❖ **Drug interactions s**

Dolutegravir (DTG) should not be co-administered with divalent cations, as these significantly reduce DTG bioavailability (by 40-75%). Magnesium, aluminum, calcium and ferrous iron should be administered 6 h before or 2 h after DTG. This interaction is linked to DTG's antiretroviral mechanism of action, which chelates the magnesium used by viral integrase as an enzymatic cofactor.

Strong enzyme inducers of CYPA3A4 and UGT1A1 reduce DTG exposure. Carbamazepine, like rifampicin, leads to a 50% reduction in DTG AUC.

DTG, on the other hand, causes metformin accumulation through inhibition of the renal transporter OCT-2. This combination must therefore be handled with caution, as it can lead to lactic acidosis, which is fatal in 50% of cases. Maximum doses (1000 mg x 3 / day) of metformin are therefore not recommended. [47].

2.7.3. Dolutegravir side effects

In clinical trials, Dolutegravir, like all integrase inhibitors, was well tolerated, generally safe and effective. However, as with any treatment, there have been adverse events of which patients taking Dolutegravir should be aware. The most frequent were

- Headaches ;
- Difficulty falling asleep ;
- Nausea ;
- Diarrhea;
- Dizzy sensation;
- Nightmare;
- Vertigo.
- Neural tube defects.

Other adverse events may be reported as Dolutegravir becomes more widely used in the community, as is the case with any new drug. [31].

2.7.4. Therapeutic perspectives s

The only solution found to date is to continue the tritherapy for life. In fact, all the antiviral drugs used to date have favored a Darwinian evolution of HIV: over time, the virus develops mutations that make it resistant to the molecules, enabling it to escape their action. Until now, these mutations have always been favorable to the virus. Dolutegravir has proved to be the first antiretroviral molecule to have the opposite effect: if mutations are selected, they are unfavorable to HIV, whose replicative capacity (known as fitness) is reduced by 80%.

If this were to be confirmed in vivo in patients not pre-treated with the integrase inhibitor, it would open up new hypotheses on site-directed mutagenesis. "If we obtain these two mutations, it's possible that the virus will be able to multiply only minimally, or not at all", says Pierre Dellamonica, Professor of Infectious Diseases at Nice University Hospital. At present, research is focused on vaccines and attempts to eradicate the virus. It is therefore legitimate to explore this new hypothesis by building up a cohort of patients treated with Dolutegravir and setting up a clinical trial of early treatment with Dolutegravir. This latter approach would make it possible to put HIV out of action while preserving the cellular immunity (CTL) developed against it, which would then be able to control HIV instead of antiretrovirals...and thus stop them [62].

3. Biological monitoring of PLWHA on treatment in Burkina Faso

Biological monitoring of HIV patients on treatment plays an essential role in the management of HIV infection. Monitoring of the treated patient allows verification of treatment tolerance through biochemical and hematological parameters [28].

Given the problems of access to biological analyses, the WHO has defined priorities between strictly essential tests, desirable tests and optional tests:

- Basic assessment strongly recommended: CBC, ALAT/ASAT, creatinine, blood sugar, pregnancy test;
- Desirable tests: bilirubinemia, lipidemia, CD4 count;
- Optional tests: plasma viral load.

These tests should be carried out at reasonable intervals of 3-6 months. Other biological tests may be carried out depending on the patient's clinical condition and the molecules used. [44].

In Burkina Faso, the follow-up schedule after initiation of treatment is as follows: M1, M3, M6 then M12 and every 6 months after the first year [9].

3.1 Investigation of blood count parameters

The haemogram measures the absolute number of cells contained per unit volume of blood [18].

3.1.1. Quantitative analysis of red blood cells

For quantitative measurements of red blood cells and their contents, the quantity of red blood cells present in a blood sample can be assessed by three measurements: the number of red blood cells, the hematocrit and the hemoglobin level.

Normal number of red blood cells

Red blood cells are anucleate, organelle-free cells containing hemoglobin. Any change in these criteria indicates a pathological phenomenon. The number of red blood cells varies with age and sex (Table VII).

Table VIII Red blood cell count by age and sex

Population	Red blood cell count (.10^{12} cells /l)
Men	4,5 à 6,2
Puberty and adult women	4 à 5,4
Child	3,6 à 5
Newborn	5 à 6

Hemoglobin level

Hemoglobin in a blood sample is measured by various methods, including the cyanmethemoglobin method, in which hemoglobin and all its derivatives are converted by a hydrocyanic acid-based reagent into cyanmethemoglobin, which is measured on a spectrophotometer at 540 nm. Results are expressed per 100 ml (dl) of blood. Table IX shows the distribution of hemoglobin levels according to sex and age.

Table IX Hemoglobin levels by age and sex

Categories	Hemoglobin level (g/dl)
Men	13 à 18
Woman	12 à 16
Child	12 à 16
Newborn	14 à 20

Red blood cell volume and content (VGM, CCMH, TCMH)

Red blood cell content depends on the amount of hemoglobin synthesized during erythropoiesis and the volume of the hematite. These are mainly assessed by calculating the so-called Wintrobe constants: mean corpuscular volume (MCV), mean corpuscular hemoglobin concentration (MCHC) and mean corpuscular hemoglobin content (MCHC).

Table X Normal values for VGM, CCMH and TCMH

Categories	VGM (fl)
	80 - 100
	CCMH (%)
Men and women	32 - 36
	TCMH (%)
	27 - 31

3.1.2. Quantitative white blood cell count

White blood cells, or leukocytes, are motile cells, all possessing organelles fundamental to animal cells, which play a defensive role in the body. Normal values are 4000 to 10000/mm3 in adults. The leukocyte formula shows the distribution of different types of white blood cells. It also checks whether the white blood cells appear normal. The five types of white blood cells and their approximate percentage in the blood are shown in the following table:

Table XI Normal values of a leukocyte formula

Category	White blood cells	Number (10^3/mm^3)
	Leukocytes	4 - 10
	Neutrophils	1,5 - 7
Men and women	Lymphocytes	1,5 - 4
	Monocytes	0,1 - 1
	Eosinophils	0,05 - 0,5
	Basophils	0,01 - 0,05

The blood of children under the age of four contains a higher percentage of lymphocytes than that of adults.

3.1.3. Quantitative platelet count

They are small, anucleated cells 2 to 4 µm in diameter, with only a few stained granules. Platelets are the main players in primary hemostasis. The most advanced electronic counters can simultaneously count red blood cells, white blood cells and platelets on the same sample. The range of normal variation is very wide (Table XI).

Table XII Normal values for blood platelets

Categories	Platelet count (10^3/mm^3)
Men and women	150- 400

3.1.4. Some pathophysiological variations in the blood count

- Anemia: defined as Hb < 13g/dl in men, and 12g/dl in women and children > 2 years.
- Moderate anemia: 7g/dl < Hb >10g/dl
- Severe anemia: Hb < 4000/mm3 of blood

- Hyperleukocytosis: hyperleukocytosis is defined as a WBC count > 10,000/mm³ blood.
- Microcytosis: defined as VGM < 80 fl in adults.
- Normocytosis: when VGM was between 80 and 100 fl in adults.
- Macrocytosis: defined by a GMV > 100fl in adults.
- Hypochromia: induced when MCHT is < 27 pg in adults.
- Mild thrombocytopenia: defined as : 100,000/mm³ < platelet count < 150,000/mm³.
- Moderate thrombocytopenia: 50,000/mm³ < platelet count < 100,000/mm³.
- Severe thrombocytopenia: platelet count 450,000/mm³.
- Lymphocytosis: When lymphocyte count > 4000/mm³ in adults;
- Lymphopenia: when lymphocyte count is < 1500/mm³.

3.2. Exploration of biochemical parameters

3.2.1. Creatininemia

Definition

Creatinine is a breakdown product of skeletal muscle creatine, which is synthesized in the liver and kidney. It is mainly eliminated by the kidneys via glomerular filtration, but also by tubular secretion (very low). It is not reabsorbed at the tubular level, making it a good indicator of glomerular function. Creatinine clearance is defined as the volume of plasma in ml completely cleared by this substance in one minute [14,26].

Dosing advantages

Serum creatinine is used as a biochemical marker of glomerular function: the simplest and most reliable, since its value is used to calculate the estimated glomerular filtration rate (GFR). It can then be used to readjust drug doses in patients. Its normal value varies according to age and sex [14,26].

Table XIII Creatinine reference values by age and sex

Categories	Creatinemia (umol/L)
Men	65 -120
Woman	50 -100
Children (4 -10 years)	30 -70
Children (10 - 14 years)	40 - 90
Newborn	60 - 90

3.2.2. Transaminases

Transaminases or aminotransferases are intracellular enzymes that catalyze the transfer of an amino group from an amino acid to an α-keto acid. There are two types of transaminase: Aspartate aminotransferase or ASAT is a glycoprotein enzyme present in the cytoplasm and mitochondria of cells in several organs, including the liver, muscles, heart, kidneys, brain and pancreas. Its elevation reflects cellular damage and is found in heart disease, hepatobiliary disorders and muscle damage. Alanine aminotransferase or ALAT is a cytosolic enzyme characteristic of the liver, and its release into the extracellular domain is certainly a sign of liver damage.

The transaminase assay is useful in :

- Cardiac pathologies (abandoned): in the case of myocardial infarction, there is an increase in ASAT, unlike ALAT, which is only slightly or not at all increased;

- Muscular pathologies: in certain myopathies, in particular progressive muscular dystrophy of the Duchenne type, which causes an increase in AST;

- Liver pathologies: ASAT and ALAT are markers of cell damage and cytolysis[7,71,73]

Table XIII shows the normal values for AST and ALT [7,71,73] :

Table XIV ASAT and ALAT reference values

Categories	ASAT (IU)	ALAT(UI)
Men and women	10 - 40	8 - 38

3.2.3. Blood glucose

Definition

Glycemia is the level of glucose in the blood. Glucose is an aldohexose with several alcohol functions and an aldehyde reducing function. It is the body's main sugar, due to its abundance and its energetic and metabolic properties, and is also an essential chemical messenger. This makes blood glucose one of the most sought-after biochemical parameters in routine and emergency care. Glucose is considered to be the almost exclusive fuel of neurons, and therefore of the brain, and of muscle during intense exertion. Any lack of blood glucose disrupts brain function. Glucose metabolism releases 4.1 kilocalories, or 17 kilojoules per gram. Some of the calories released for cellular activity or muscular work appear in the form of heat, which helps maintain body temperature [41,49,51,52].

Physiological regulation

Blood sugar regulation is part of the process of maintaining homeostasis within the body. It involves several systems: organs and metabolic pathways. It involves several organs, in particular the liver, which is the key organ in glycemic regulation via three mechanisms:

glycogenogenesis, glycogenolysis and gluconeogenesis; adipose tissue, the second reservoir of carbohydrate storage; muscles, which can store glucose in the form of glycogen; and the kidney and interstitial environment, which are involved in pathological situations. [41,49,51,52].

Hormonal regulation

The main hormones involved in this regulation are :

- Insulin: the only hypoglycemic hormone secreted by the β-cells of the islets of Langerhans, it acts primarily by inhibiting glycogenolysis and neoglucogenesis and stimulating glycogenogenesis and glycolysis.

- Glucagon: a hyperglycemic hormone produced by the α cells of the islets of Langerhans, its action counteracts that of insulin. Other hormones, such as adrenalin, cortisol, growth hormone and thyroid hormones, also have a hyperglycemic effect. [41,49,51,52].

Nerve regulation

The sympathetic system plays a crucial role during sudden hypoglycemia, while the parasympathetic system is involved in coordinating hyper- and hypoglycemic responses. [41,49,51,52].

Clinical benefits

Glycemia is the central parameter in the investigation of disorders of carbohydrate metabolism, particularly in the screening of diabetes. It is also of interest in the biological assessment of certain pancreatic, adrenal, pituitary and thyroid disorders, as well as in the monitoring of treatment with corticoids and certain diuretics. Table XIV shows normal blood glucose values [41,49,51,52].

Table XV Normal blood glucose values by age

Fasting blood glucose	mmol/L
Newborn	1,66 - 3,32
Children / Adults	3,9 - 6,1

3.2.4. Amylasemia

Amylase is an enzyme found in pancreatic juice and saliva, which converts starch and glycogen into dextrins and maltose during intestinal digestion. Inflammation or obstruction of the salivary gland ducts increases blood levels and urinary excretion of amylase. Amylase levels are useful in diagnosing pancreatitis. It is elevated in acute and chronic pancreatitis, pancreatic cancer, pseudocysts of the pancreas, occlusion of pancreatic ducts, perforated stomach ulcers, acute appendicitis, damage to the parotid glands, certain drugs, etc.

In acute pancreatitis, serum amylase rises after a few hours and normalizes within 2 to 3 days.

In chronic pancreatitis, amylasemia is sometimes moderately increased during painful attacks: ulcer perforations, cholecystitis, small bowel occlusions, mesenteric infarction [19,29,32,70].

Normal values for amylasemia are given in the following table [20] :

Table XVI Variation in amylasemia

Amylasemia (at 37°C)	IU/L
Newborns and infants	≤32
Child	≤85
Adult	≤85

PART TWO: OUR STUDY

OBJECTIVES

II. OBJECTIVES

1. General objective

To study the evolution of biological parameters of antiretroviral therapeutic protocols including Dolutegravir in people living with HIV (PLHIV) followed in 2022 in the dermatology and internal medicine departments of the CHU-YO.

2. Specific objectives

1. To describe the socio-demographic characteristics of HIV patients undergoing DTG in the dermatology and internal medicine departments of CHU-YO ;
2. Identify DTG-based ARV protocols used in the dermatology and internal medicine departments of CHU-YO ;
3. To determine the evolution of hematological parameters of antiretroviral protocols including DTG in HIV PLHIV in the dermatology and internal medicine departments of the CHU YO ;
4. To determine the evolution of biochemical parameters of antiretroviral protocols including DTG in HIV patients in the dermatology and internal medicine departments of CHU-YO.

METHODOLOGY

III. METHODOLOGY

1. Scope of the study

Our study was conducted at the Centre Hospitalo-Universitaire Yalgado OUEDRAOGO (CHU-YO), in the dermatology and internal medicine departments.

2. Type of study and study period

This was a cross-sectional study with retrospective data collection. HIV patients on DTG treated in dermatology and internal medicine departments between December 2020 and December 2023 were included in the data collection.

3. Study population

Our study population included all people living with HIV followed up in the dermatology and internal medicine departments of CHU-YO during the study period.

3.1 Inclusion criteria

All patients will be included in our study:

- Follow-up with an ARV protocol including Dolutegravir during the study period;

- Having a file with at least one biological examination completed at initiation and after 6 months of treatment during the study period.

3.2 Non-inclusion criteria

Not included in our study:

All patients not on antiretroviral protocol including dolutegravir;

Patients with no usable clinical records.

4.   Sampling

This was an exhaustive sample of HIV patients meeting our inclusion criteria. In fact, our study sample included all HIV-positive patients on an ARV protocol including DTG, in the dermatology and internal medicine departments, during the period from December 2020 to December 2022, and who underwent biological examinations at initiation and then after 6 months of treatment.

5. Collecting data

Our data were collected using a data collection form, the source of which was the PLHIV's medical records.

6. Study variables

The study variables were :

- **Socio-demographic characteristics of HIV patients** : age, sex, occupation, marital status
- **Biological characteristics of** PLWHA: biochemical parameters (creatininemia, glycemia, transaminases, cholesterolemia, triglycerides, HDL, LDL, amylasemia), blood count.
- **Therapeutic features:** therapeutic protocols, treatment compliance.

7. Data analysis and interpretation
- The data was entered using Epi-info 7.2.5.0 software;
- Analysis was performed using Microsoft Excel 2020.

8. Ethical and deontological considerations
- Authorization from the CEO of CHU-YO and the heads of the dermatology and internal medicine departments was required;

- Data was collected anonymously using the data collection form, in order to preserve patient privacy and confidentiality.

RESULTS

IV. RESULTS

For our study, out of a total of 882 patient files under protocol including DTG, we selected 151 patients whose follow-up biological examinations were carried out at treatment initiation and again after 6 months, and correctly recorded in the clinical record. The following flow chart shows our recruitment procedure.

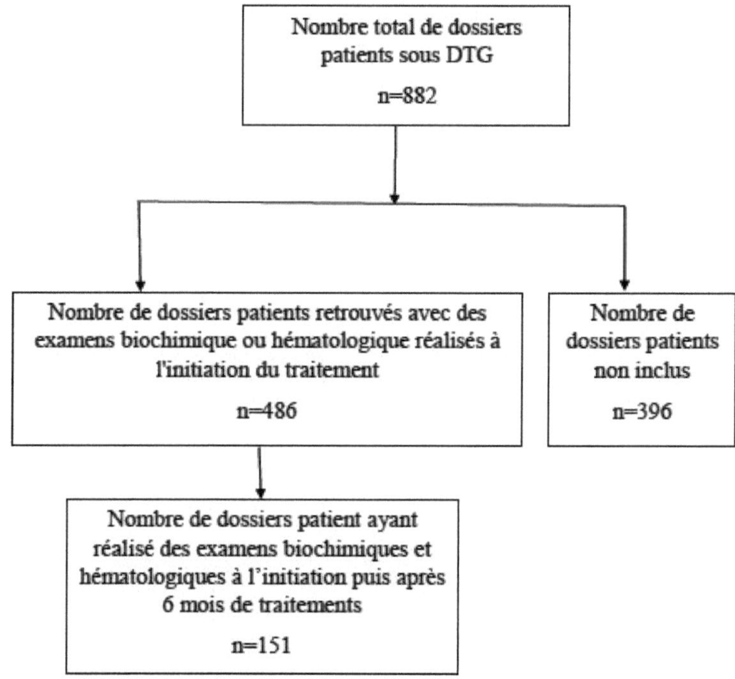

Figure 2 Flow chart

1. Socio-demographic data

1.1. Age and gender

The age and gender of DTG patients are summarized in Table XVI.

Table XVII Distribution of patients according to socio-demographic variables.

Age ranges	Number (n)	Percentage (%)
25-49 years	91	60,3
50 and over	51	33,7
15-24 years	9	6
Sex		
Female	86	57,0
Male	65	43,0
Total (N)	**151**	**100**

91 patients, or 60.3% of cases, were aged between [25-49 years].
Female patients numbered 86 (57%), with a sex ratio of 0.76 men to 1 woman.

1.2. Socio-professional status

The socio-professional status of the patients included in our study is shown in Table XVII.

Table XVIII Distribution of patients according to socio-professional status nel

Socio-professional status	Number of employees (n)	Percentage (%)
Housewives	31	20,53
Private-sector employee	22	14,57
Retailer	20	13,24
Artisan	19	12,58
Civil servant	17	11,27
Student	14	9,27
Retired	11	7,28
Cultivator	9	5,96
Liberal profession	8	5,3
Total (N)	**151**	**100**

Housewives accounted for 20.53% of cases in our study.

1.3. Marital status

The marital status of our patients is shown in Table XVIII.

Painting XIX Summary of marital status of PLHIV on DTG

Marital status	Number (n)	Percentage (%)
Married	64	42,38
Single	47	31,12
Widow	20	13,24
Divorced	12	7,95
Concubinage	8	5,3

Total (N)	151	100

Married people accounted for 42.38% of cases.

1.4. Residence

Residence	Number of employees (n)	Percentage (%)
Ouagadougou	129	85,3%
Outside Ouagadougou	22	14,7%

Patients residing in Ouagadougou accounted for 85.3% of cases.

2. Frequency of use of ARV protocols including DTG

The frequency of ARV treatment protocols including DTG is shown in Table XIX.

Table XX Frequency of different DTG-based ARV protocols

DTG-based protocol	Workforce	Percentage (%)	Total (n)
TDF/3TC/DTG (TLD)	138	91,4%	151
ABC/3TC+DTG (ALD)	13	8,6%	151

The TDF/3TC/DTG (TLD) protocol was found in 91.4% of patients on ARV protocols including DTG.

3. Treatment compliance

Compliance with HIV treatment is shown in Table XX.

Table XXI Summary of therapeutic compliance

Observance (patient compliance with prescribed treatment) N=151	Number of employees (n)	Percentage
Good compliance	145	96,0%
Poor compliance	6	4,0%
Total	**151**	**100%**

Compliance was good in 96% of patients.

4. Types of HIV treated with DTG

The different types of HIV encountered in our study are shown in Table XXI :

Table XXII Distribution of HIV types encountered

Type of HIV	Workforce(n)	Percentage (%)
HIV 1	144	95,4%
HIV 2	2	1,3%
HIV1 + 2	5	3,3%

HIV type 1 was found in 95.4% of patients.

5. Paraclinical data

5.1. Tests performed

The following table shows the distribution of patients according to the examinations prescribed and performed:

Table XXIII Tests performed

Tests performed	Numbers (n=151)	Percentages (%)
Creatininemia	73	48,34
Blood count	69	45,7

	64	42,38
Blood glucose	64	42,38
ALAT/ASAT	59	39,07
Amylasemia	12	7,95
Cholesterol	9	5,96
CRP	4	2,65

The rates of creatinine and blood count were 48.34% and 45.70% respectively.

5.2. Blood count

The results of blood count parameters obtained at initiation (T1) and after 6 months (T2) of treatment are shown in Table XXIII.

Table XXIV Blood count

Hematological parameters (n=69)	Averages $(T_1 - T_2)$	Work force $(T_1 - T_2)$	Percentages (%) $(T_1 - T_2)$
HB level (g/dL)	12,1 - 13,32		
Anemia		41 - 14	59,42 - 20,29
Normal		25 - 52	36,23 - 75,36
Hb >		3 - 3	4,35 - 4,35
Leukocyte (cells/mm^3)	270653,16 - 6049,17		
Leukopenia		25 - 3	36,23 - 4,64
Normal		40 - 66	57,97 - 95,36
Hyperleukocytosis		4 - 0	5,8 - 0

	Averages	Workforce	Percentages
Lymphocytes (cells/mm)³	2208,78 - 2333,63		
Lymphopenia		20 - 0	28,98 - 0
Normal		44 - 69	63,77 - 100
Lymphocytosis		5 - 0	7,25 - 0
Platelet (cells/mm)³	226592,85 - 367166,67		
Thrombocytopenia		12 - 10	17,39 - 14,49
Normal		57 - 56	82,61 - 81,16
Thrombocytosis		0 - 3	0 - 4,35

5.3. Biochemical parameters

The various biochemical parameter results obtained at treatment initiation
(T1) and after 6 months (T2) are shown in Table XXIV.

Table XXV Biochemical parameters

Parameters	Averages (T_1-T_2)	Workforce (T_1-T_2)	Percentages (%) (T_1-T_2)
Creatininemia (μ mol/L) n= 73	69,33 - 83,48		
Normal creatinine		70 - 66	95,89 - 90,41
Hyper-creatininemia		1- 6	1,37 - 8,22
Decreased creatinine		2 - 1	2,74 - 1,37
Blood glucose (mmol/L) n= 67	5,17 - 5,51		
Hypoglycemia		4 - 2	5,97 - 2,98

Normal blood glucose		50 - 55	74,63 - 82,1
Hyperglycemia		13 - 10	19,4 - 14,92
ALAT (UI/L) n= 59	31,7 - 40,42		
ALAT normal		50 - 46	84,75 - 77,97
ALAT increased		9 - 13	15,25 - 22,03
AST (UI/L) n= 59	38,71 - 45,93		
ASAT normal		37 - 45	62,71 - 76,27
ASAT increased		22 - 14	37,29 - 23,73

DISCUSSION

V. DISCUSSION

1. Study limitations and constraints

Our study is a retrospective study conducted over a two-year period, from December 2020 to December 2022. It has limitations that are inherent in most retrospective studies, namely:

- The retrospective nature of the study,
- Our sample size ;
- Incomplete clinical records;
- Failure to carry out prescribed examinations ;
- Patients' failure to keep follow-up appointments;
- Control examinations are carried out every six months;
- Patient files with incomplete or inconsistent information.
- The follow-up time (6 months) is short and does not enable us to better assess the evolution of short- and long-term adverse biological effects.

Our study has nevertheless produced results that call for comment and discussion. The analyses have taken these limitations into account, as have the interpretations and conclusions based on the results obtained.

2. Socio-demographic characteristics of patients

In our study, the mean age of patients was 45 years, with extremes of 17 and 89 years. The 25 to 49 age group was the most represented. Our results are similar to those of Karfo et *al.* in Burkina Faso in 2018, who found an average age of 44 years, a predominance of the 25 to 54 age group, with extremes of 16 and 81 years. [37]. The representativeness of this age bracket is explained by the fact that it corresponds to that of maximum sexual activity exposing to the risks of transmission of sexually transmitted infections. The predominance of heterosexual transmission in tropical regions, particularly in sub-Saharan Africa, may explain the prevalence of the disease in this age group. [4,45].

Female patients predominated, with a sex ratio of 0.76 in favor of females. In fact, 57% of patients were female, compared with 43% male. The trend towards feminization of HIV infection has been reported by several authors [15,40,66]. This result could be explained by the higher prevalence of HIV observed among women in Burkina Faso, but also by women's increasing access to screening thanks to prevention of mother-to-child transmission (PMTCT) programs.

Of the patients in the study, 42.38% were married. These results are close to those of Issa KABORE in Burkina Faso, who reported 60.90%. [35]. Stigmatization and denial of the disease in couples could explain the predominance of married people. Polygamy is also common in our country.

The majority of patients included in our study lived in the city of Ouagadougou (85.3%). This could be explained by the fact that the study was carried out in Ouagadougou.

3. Biological and therapeutic data

3.1 Frequency of different DTG-based ARV protocols

In our study, the TLD protocol was the most common, with a rate of 91.4%, compared with 8.6% for the ABC+3TC+DTG protocol. These results are similar to those of Niambele and Bouarés, who found 71.1% and 98.6% respectively for the TLD protocol [5,63]. This may be explained by the application of new WHO recommendations for HIV management, according to which all PLWHA should be reversed to the TLD protocol.

3.2. Treatment compliance

Therapeutic compliance is essential for the success of ARV treatment.

In our study, compliance was good in 96% of our patients. Saliou [61]Goita [27] and Traoré N'Z [69] found 89.3%, 86.1% and 66.67% good compliance respectively. This may be explained by the simplicity of the TLD protocol treatment regimens.

3.3. Types of HIV affected by DTG-based treatment

In our study, 95.4% of patients were of the HIV1 type. Similar results were shown in the studies by DIALLO A [17] entitled "Antiretroviral treatment adherence among adult patients living with HIV followed at the support and counseling unit of the reference health center of commune vi of the Bamako district" and of DENE E.K. [16] entitled "Suivi des paramètres biologiques des PVVIH sous traitement ARV à l'EPH de Gao", with rates of 97% and 95.1% respectively. This could be explained by the fact that HIV1 is the most prevalent in West Africa and worldwide.

3.4. Tests performed

Biochemical tests were the most frequently prescribed and performed in our study (57.6%), led by creatinine levels (83.91%).

These tests enable us to assess the patient's general condition, as well as the biological tolerance of the current treatment. They are therefore very important in the therapeutic follow-up of patients.

Serum creatinine is the most widely prescribed and performed test in our case, due to its availability and accessibility. Serum creatinine is also used as a biochemical marker of glomerular function: the simplest and most reliable, since its value is used to calculate the estimated glomerular filtration rate (GFR). [26]. This test can therefore be used to determine the most appropriate treatment protocol for the patient.

3.5. Hematological characteristics

3.5.1. Hemoglobin (Hb) level

In our study, 59.42% of patients had moderate anemia (7g/dL < Hb level <10g/dL) at treatment initiation. This rate regressed after 6 months of treatment to 20.29%. We also obtained mean hemoglobin levels that rose from 12.1 at initiation to 13.32g/dL after 6 months on DTG. These results are similar to those of the University of Bamako, by Keita et al in 2023, with an increase in hemoglobin levels after 6 months of triple therapy [39]. Also, Karfo et *al.* found a regression in the rate of anemia, and the mean hemoglobin level rose from 10.5g/dL at M0 to 12.53 g/dL at M12 [37]. This may be explained by the fact that our sample does not comprise naive PLWHA.

3.5.2. Leukocytes

White blood cell count results showed a normal leukocyte count of 57.97% at DTG initiation. This rate improved to 95.36% after 6 months of DTG treatment. This result could be explained by the efficacy of DTG-containing protocols.

3.5.3. Inserts

Platelets were normal in 82.61% of cases at initiation of ART including DTG. After 6 months of treatment with DTG, normal platelet counts varied little (81.16%). Thrombocytopenia was observed in (17.39%) of cases at initiation and regressed by M6 (14.49). These results are similar to those of Edith, who found (82.9%) normal platelets [36]. In contrast,

Karfo et *al.* found thrombocytopenia in 12.5% of cases, which did not progress significantly [37].

3.6. Biochemical characteristics

3.6.1. Creatininemia

Creatinine levels in our study were normal, ranging from 95.89% to 90.41%, respectively at treatment initiation and after 6 months. However, mean creatinine levels changed from 69.33 to 83.48µ mol/L. These values remain normal, however. These results are similar to those of Keita et *al.*[39] and BREMA [6] who found respectively 68% and 95.3% of cases with normal creatinine levels. The increase in mean creatinine levels at M6 on ART could probably be due to the side effects of Tenofovir present in the TLD [23,74].

3.6.2. Blood glucose

In our study, 74.63% of cases had normal blood glucose levels at treatment initiation. This rate improved significantly to 82.1% after 6 months of DTG treatment. Hyperglycemia was observed in 19.4% of cases at initiation, then regressed at M6 (14.92% of cases). This could be explained by the fact that these patients had hyperglycemia prior to DTG use. These results are similar to those of a study conducted in Togo in 2019, which found 12.4% hyperglycemia in patients on protease inhibitors (PIs) [3]. Mean blood glucose values varied little (5.17 - 5.51) and remained normal.

3.6.3. Transaminases

ALT levels were normal in 77.97% of cases after 6 months of DTG treatment. It should be noted that this level was slightly lower than at baseline (84.75%). We also observed an increase in mean ALT levels from 31.7IU/L to 40.42IU/L after 6 months of treatment.

We also noted an increase in the average ASAT level from 38.71 to 45.93IU/L, thus exceeding normal values (< 40IU/L).

These findings suggest that DTG-based protocols may have an impact on transaminases, particularly ASAT levels. These results are similar to those of Maggi et *al.* who also found an increase in transaminases under a regimen based on a non-nucleoside reverse transcriptase inhibitor (Doravirine) [46].

3.6.4. Lipid profile

The analysis of lipid profiles (triglyceride, cholesterol, HDL and LDL levels) among these patients could not be carried out either due to insufficient data or the absence of a valid pair. In fact, very few patients had undergone these tests, and in those cases where they had, there were almost no controls at M6 (after 6 months of treatment) to enable us to monitor their progress over time.

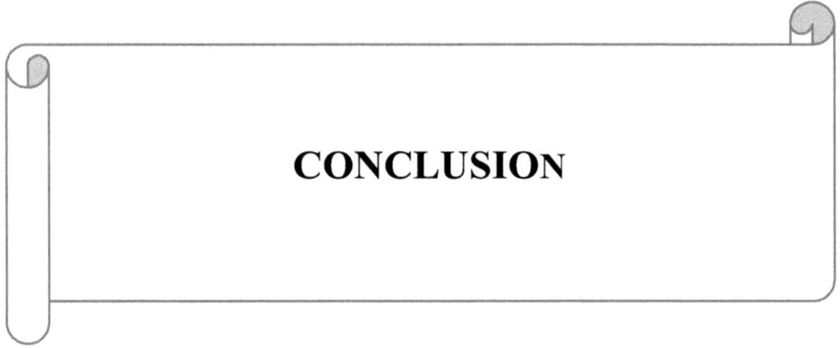

CONCLUSION

CONCLUSION

In our study, the average age of patients was 45, with a predominance of females. The TLD protocol was the most recurrent, and HIV type 1 was in the majority. Access to investigative tools for biological monitoring of HIV patients remains a handicap in our active file. Nonetheless, this study revealed that protocols including DTG had a significant influence on biological parameters, although these remained normal for most of the parameters studied. Indeed, according to our study, DTG-based protocols led to an abnormal increase in transaminase (ASAT) levels.

SUGGESTIONS

SUGGESTIONS

In the light of the study we have carried out, we would like to make a few suggestions for the attention of the various healthcare players in our country:

To the Permanent Secretary of CNLS/IST :

- Supply healthcare facilities with ARV molecules (TAF) to avoid renal toxicity;
- Follow the update of the new protocols for the management of HIV patients recommended by the WHO.

To the General Manager of CHU-YO   :

- Promote the introduction of a modern archiving system;
- Set up a computerized medical records system

To the head of the ARV dispensing unit :

Carry out a prospective study of biological parameters in HIV patients on ART including DTG.

To caregivers:

- Prescribing lipid profiles;
- Ensure that patient examinations are correctly recorded in the clinical record and that the clinical record is properly maintained.

People living with HIV:

- Adhere to ARV treatment and carry out all prescribed tests.

REFERENCES

REFERENCES

1. **ActionTreatments**. Injectable antiretrovirals: more than just a new mode of administration? [Internet]. Actions Traitements, association de patients VIH et co-infections. 2022 [cited 4 Feb 2024]. Available from: https://actions-traitements.org/antiretroviraux-en-injection-plus-quun-nouveau-mode-administration/

2. **Adams JL, Greener BN, Kashuba AD**. Pharmacology of HIV integrase inhibitors. Curr Opin HIV AIDS. 2012;7(5):390.

3. **Agbeko DK, Toyi T, Lihanimpo D, Dzidzonu NK, Laconi K, Abago B, Awalou DM**. Lipid and carbohydrate disorders at cardiovascular risk in people living with human immunodeficiency virus under antiretroviral treatment: case of the medical care center of the NGO Espoir-Vie-Togo in Lomé. Pan Afr Med J. 2019;34(1):89.

4. **Aubry P**. Infection par le VIH/Sida et tropiques Actualités. Méd Trop. 2012;34(2):74.

5. **Bouaré BS**. Etudes des paramètres clinico-biologiques des patients adultes initiés aux traitements antirétroviral du 1er janvier 2017 au 31 Décembre 2018 à l'hôpital Nianankoro Fomba (HNF) de Ségou [Thèse de doctorat en medecine]. Université des Sciences, des Techniques et des Technologies de Bamako; 2020.

6. **Bréma C**. Suivi du bilan biologique chez les personnes vivant avec le VIH et le SIDA sous traitement antirétroviral au CESAC de Bamako du 1er janvier 2009 au 31 janvier 2010 Bamako. 2010. Accessed August. 2017;2(130):107.

7. **CHI-PANG W.** Hepatocellular carcinoma risk prediction model for the general population: the predictive power of transaminases. J Natl Cancer Inst. 2012;3(145):1599-1611p.

8. **ClinicalTrials**. Mode of action of antiretroviral therapies [Internet]. VIH Clic. 2014 [cited Sep 12, 2023]. Available from: https://vihclic.fr/antiretro-viraux/mode-action-physiopathologie-traitements-antiretroviraux/

9. **CNLS-IST**. Normes et protocoles de prises en charge des personnes infectées et affectées par le VIH/SIDA au BURKINA FASO. Ouagadougou 2021.

10. **CNLS-IST**. Rapport d'activité sur la riposte au SIDA du Burkina Faso. GLOBAL AIDS MONOTORING (GAM) 2019.

11. **CNLS-IST, CMLS/Santé**. Normes et protocoles de prise en charge médicale des personnes vivant avec le VIH au BURKINA FASO 2009.

12. **Communications**. New HIV drugs! - Capsid inhibitors [Internet]. PVSQ. 2023 [cited Feb 22, 2024]. Available from: https://pvsq.org/2023/inhibiteurs-capside/

13. **Congress US**. United States leadership against HIV/AIDS, tuberculosis, and malaria act of 2003. Public Law. 2003;(108-25).

14. **Delatour V, Lalere B, Dumont G, Hattchouel J-M, Froissart M, De Graeve J, Vaslin-Reimann S**. Development of a reference method for creatinine determination to improve diagnosis and monitoring of renal failure. Rev Fr Métrologie. 2011;(26).

15. **Dembele E**. Identification of factors associated with ARV therapeutic failure in patients living with HIV1 followed at the FOUSSEYNI DAOU hospital in Kayes. Bamako Univ Sci Tech Technol Bamako. 2018;138(2):129.

16. **Déné EK**. Suivi des paramètres biologiques des PVVIH sous traitement ARV à l'EPH de GAO. Thèse d'Etat en pharmacie N° 154, Université de Bamako, Mali; 2011.

17. **Diallo A**. Etude de l'observance aux traitements antirétroviraux chez les patients "Populations Clés" suivis à la clinique les Halles de ARCAD-Santé Plus de Juin 2018 à Mai 2019. Thèse d'Etat en pharmacie N° 122, Université des Sciences, des Techniques et des Technologies de Bamako, Mali; 2021.

18. **Donadieu J, Leblanc T, Meunier BB, Barkaoui M, Fenneteau O, Bertrand Y, Maier-Redelsperger M, Micheau M, Stephan JL, Phillipe N**. Analysis of risk factors for myelodysplasias, leukemias and death from infection among patients with congenital neutropenia. Experience of the French Severe Chronic Neutropenia Study Group. haematologica. 2005;90(1):45-53.

19. **Durand H, Biclet P**. Dictionnaire des examens biologiques et investigations paracliniques. Pari: Doin; 2015.

20. **Emélie Kalifa**. Amylase: Analysis, Blood or Urine examination, Results. 2015.

21. **IN DANGER: UNAIDS**. Global AIDS Report Update 2022. 2022.

22. **Fongoro PS, Traore DAA, Sidibe DY, Oumar DAA, Dao PS**. Adverse effects of ARVs in HIV-infected patients at Sikasso regional hospital and Sikasso CERKES. 2012;13(2):86.

23. **Gallant JE, Parish MA, Keruly JC, Moore RD**. Changes in renal function associated with tenofovir disoproxil fumarate treatment, compared with nucleoside reverse-transcriptase inhibitor treatment. Clin Infect Dis. 2005;40(8):1194-8.

24. **Ghosn J**. Dolutegravir: a new integrase inhibitor in the anti-HIV therapeutic arsenal. J Anti-Infect. 2015;17(3):111-4.

25. **Global HIV**. AIDS statistics-Fact sheet. Unaids Org. 2021; 86p

26. **Godin-Ribuot PD**. Measurement of renal function: renal clearance. 2011;Grenoble 1(35):139.

27. **Goita Z**. Observance of ARV treatment among HIV+ patients at the Kénédougou S solidarité reference center in Sikasso. These Pharmacie N° 122, Bamako, Mali; 2008.

28. **Greder Belan A, Chaplain C, Boussairi A**. Biological monitoring of HIV infection in adults. Immuno-Anal Biol Spéc. 2008;23(2):95-102.

29. **Hassan T, Mikhail N, Cappell MS**. Extrapulmonic Pneumocystis carinii infection at a porta hepatis lymph node. 1992;3(27):134.

30. **HIV/AIDS (UNAIDS) UNP on**. Global HIV & AIDS Statistics-2020 Fact Sheet. 2020.

31. **Hosein SR**. Fact sheet [Internet]. CATIE - Canada's source for HIV and hepatitis C information. 2018. Available at:

https://www.catie.ca/fr/education-publications-et-sites-web-publications-pour-les-prestataires-de-services/feuillets

32. **Ilboudo B**. L'Amylasémie au cours de l'infection à VIH : à propos de 143 cas colligés au Centre de Traitement Ambulatoire (CTA) de Ouagadougou. Thèse d'Etat en Médecine N° 33, Ouagadougou, Burkina Faso; 2004.

33. **Iyidogan P, Anderson KS**. Current perspectives on HIV-1 antiretroviral drug resistance. Viruses. 2014;6(10):4095-139.

34. **Jordheim LP, Durantel D, Zoulim F, Dumontet C**. Advances in the development of nucleoside and nucleotide analogues for cancer and viral diseases. Nat Rev Drug Discov. 2013;12(6):447-64.

35. **Kabore I**. Etude des facteurs pronostiques du traitement antirétroviral de deuxième ligne contenant de l'abacavir chez les patients vivant avec le VIH. Thèse d'Etat en Médecine N° 161, Ouagadougou, Burkina Faso; 2022.

36. **Karakodjo DE**. Suivi des paramètres biologiques des PVVIH sous traitement ARV à l'EPH de Gao. 2011;13(1):19-28.

37. **Karfo R, Kabré E, Coulibaly L, Diatto G, Sakandé J, Sangaré L**. Evolution des paramètres biochimiques et hématologiques chez les personnes vivant avec le VIH SIDA sous traitement antirétroviral au Centre Médical du Camp General Aboubacar Sangoule Lamizana (CMCGASL). Pan Afr Med J. 2018;29(1):1-7.

38. **Keita A**. Management of HIV-1 infection in developing countries: diagnostic aspects and immunovirological evaluation of therapeutic efficacy in blood and mucosal compartments. 2018;3(128):195.

39. **Keita A.** Suivi biologique des personnes vivant avec le VIH sous traitement antirétroviral au service des maladies infectieuses et tropicales et au laboratoire du CHU de Point Gde 2020 à 2022. 12(1):28-35.

40. **Konou AA, Dagnra AY, Vidal N, Salou M, Adam Z, Singo-Tokofai A, Delaporte E, Prince-David M, Peeters M.** Alarming rates of virological failure and drug resistance in patients on long-term antiretroviral treatment in routine HIV clinics in Togo. AIDs. 2015;29(18):2527-30.

41. **Laboratoires Merck Génériques/Mylan, Société Française de Biologie Clinique, Section G de l'Ordre des pharmaciens.** Guide des examens biologiques | GUID-EXAM-FEV08 guidebio150x210decembre2007 18/01/08 16:19 Page 68.

42. **Launay O.** Thérapeutiques antirétrovirales: principes du traitement de l'infection par le VIH. Presse Médicale. June 1, 2008;37(6, Part 2):1022-32.

43. **EDLLC, HIV SC, IST SE.** Plan de mise en oeuvre des directives nationales pour la prévention et le traitement du VIH au BURUNDI. Burundi; 2020.

44. **WHO, World Health Organization.** WHO consolidated guidelines on the use of antiretroviral drugs for the treatment and prevention of HIV infections. 2013.

45. **Lozes E, Ahoussinou C, Djikpo MAT, Dahouegnon E, Ahossouhe N, Acoty A, Souza C de.** Variability of CD4 lymphocyte count and viral load in people living with HIV under

antiretroviral treatment: case of the Hôpital Saint Jean De Dieu de Tanguieta (Benin). Int J Biol Chem Sci. 2012;117(2):650-6.

46. **Maggi P, Ricci ED, Cicalini S, Pellicanò GF, Celesia BM, Vichi F, Cascio A, Sarchi E, Orofino G, Squillace N, Madeddu G, De Socio GV, Bargiacchi O, Molteni C, Masiello A, Saracino A, Menzaghi B, Falasca K, Taramasso L, Di Biagio A, Bonfanti P**. Lipids and transaminase elevations in ARV-experienced PLWH switching to a doravirine-based regimen from rilpivirine or other regimens. BMC Infect Dis. 14 Apr 2023;23(1):227.

47. **Metsu D**. Intérêt de l'exploration de la forme libre du dolutegravir, du darunavir et de l'atazanavir chez les patients VIH [PhD Thesis]. [France]: Université de Toulouse, Université Toulouse III-Paul Sabatier; 2019.

48. **Michaud G**. Approach for the diastereoselective synthesis of □-nucleoside analogues and synthesis of new C2'-deoxy nucleoside analogues.

49. **MONTJAUX N., BOSSARD G**. "Hypoglycemia in the newborn at or near term". 2012. 3-10p. Hôp Enfants Toulouse Cent Hosp Cahors. 2012;2(58):3-10p.

50. **MSHP, CNLS-IST, (Ministère la Santé du Burkina Faso, Conseil National de lutte contre le VIH/SIDA et les IST)**. Normes et protocoles de prise en charges médicales des personnes vivant avec le VIH au Burkina Faso. 6th Edition; June 2021.226p.

51. **Njikeutchi DFN**. Contribution à l'établissement des valeurs de référence de paramètres biologiques chez le burkinabé adulte: évaluation de cinq constituants biochimiques au service de chimie

biologie du Centre Hospitalier Universitaire Yalgado Ouédraogo (CHU-YO) à Ouagadougou. 2003;126(2):130.

52. **NUMBER A.** Suivi de la qualité de dosage de la glycemie, de la creatininemie et de l'uremie au laboratoire de biochimie du center hospitalier universitaire pediatrique charles de gaulle. Thesis in pharmacy, thesis N° 199, Joseph KI-ZERBO University, Burkina Faso; 2014.

53. **WHO.** WHO recommends dolutegravir as the preferred HIV treatment option in all populations [Internet]. 2019 [cited August 29, 2022]. Available from: https://www.who.int/fr/news/item/22-07-2019-who-recommends-dolutegravir-as-preferred-hiv-treatment-option-in-all-populations

54. **OMS/CDS/VIH.** Update of recommendations on first- and second-line antiretroviral regimens [Internet]. 2019 [cited 6 Feb 2024]. Available from: https://www.who.int/publications-detail-redirect/WHO-CDS-HIV-19.15

55. **WHO/HIV-AIDS.** Key benchmarks on HIV/AIDS [Internet]. [cited 1 Sep 2023]. Available from: https://www.who.int/fr/news-room/fact-sheets/detail/hiv-aids

56. **UNAIDS.** UNAIDS HIV treatment [Internet]. 2020. Available at: https://www.unaids.org/fr/topic/treatment

57. **UNAIDS.** New UNAIDS report shows it is possible to end AIDS by 2030 and outlines the way forward [Internet]. 2023. Available at: https://www.unaids.org/fr/resources/presscentre/pressreleaseandstatementarchive/2023/july/unaids-global-aids-update

58. **UNAIDS**. The Joint United Nations Programme on HIV/AIDS. Fact Sheet - Latest statistics on the state of the AIDS epidemic_UNAIDS_FactSheet_en. 2023.

59. **Rosenbach KA, Allison R, Nadler JP**. Daily dosing of highly active antiretroviral therapy. Clin Infect Dis. 2002;34(5):686-92.

60. **Saint Blaise**. The AIDS epidemic in ten key dates [Internet]. ladepeche.fr. 2021. Available at: https://www.ladepeche.fr/2021/06/07/lepidemie-de-sida-en-dix-dates-cles-9591762.php

61. **Saliou M**. Suivi clinique et biologique des patients sous antirétroviraux à l'hôpital du point G. Thèse d'Etat en Medecine N° 35, Bamako, Mali; 2005.

62. **Samaké GM**. Evaluation of the therapeutic success of an antiretroviral strategy involving dolutegravir administered in HIV-infected patients followed at the USAC of the CSRef of commune VI of the District of Bamako. PhD Thesis, USTTB, Mali; 2023.

63. **Saran MNM**. Verification of HIV type in patients on Antiretrovirals at the Infectious Diseases Department of CHU Point G, Bamako, Mali. 2019;166(3):88.

64. **SP/CNLS-IST, Conseil National de Lutte contre le sida et les IST**. Cadre Stratégique de lutte contre le VIH, le Sida et les infections sexuellement transmissibles 2011-2015 (final document). Ouagadougou: 2022.

65. **SP/CNLS-IST, Conseil National de Lutte contre le sida et les IST**. Rapport d'activité sur la riposte au SIDA au Burkina Faso-

GAM [Internet]. 2019. Available at:
https://www.unaids.org/sites/default/files/country/documents/BFA_
2019_countryreport.pdf

66. **Ssempijja V, Nakigozi G, Chang L, Gray R, Wawer M, Ndyanabo A, Kasule J, Serwadda D, Castelnuovo B, Hoog A van't**. Rates of switching to second-line antiretroviral therapy and impact of delayed switching on immunologic, virologic, and mortality outcomes among HIV-infected adults with virologic failure in Rakai, Uganda. BMC Infect Dis. 2017;17:1-10.

67. **Taburet A-M, Paci-Bonaventure S, Peytavin G, Molina J-M**. Once-daily administration of antiretrovirals: pharmacokinetics of emerging therapies. Clin Pharmacokinet. 2003;42:1179-91.

68. **Tan Q, Zhu Y, Li J, Chen Z, Han GW, Kufareva I, Li T, Ma L, Fenalti G, Li J**. Structure of the CCR5 chemokine receptor-HIV entry inhibitor maraviroc complex. Science. 2013;341(6152):1387-90.

69. **Touré M**. Suivi cliniques, biologiques et thérapeutiques des personnes vivant avec le VIH sous ARV de Janvier 2018 à Décembre 2019 à l'USAC du CS Réf CVI Bamako. 2023;54(2):118.

70. **Weil JH, Boulanger J, Chambon P, Dubertret G, Gautheron D, Kedinger C, Lazdunski M, Montreuil J, Patte JC, Rebel G**. Biochimie générale 7th edition. Masson; 2000.

71. **WILKINSON J, BARON N, MOSS W, WALKER P**. Standardization of clinical enzyme assays: a reference method for aspartate and alanine transaminases. Natl Libr Med 1972. 25(11):940-4.

72. **Woollard SM, Kanmogne GD**. Maraviroc: a review of its use in HIV infection and beyond. Drug Des Devel Ther. 2015;5447-68.

73. **YATSIDIS H**. Measurement of transaminases in serum. ED Naturebriefing 1960. 13(1):79-80.

74. **Zimmermann AE, Pizzoferrato T, Bedford J, Morris A, Hoffman R, Braden G**. Tenofovir-Associated Acute and Chronic Kidney Disease: A Case of Multiple Drug Interactions. Clin Infect Dis. 2006;42(2):283-90.

APPENDICES

APPENDICES

Data collection form :

		M1...	M2...	M3	M4
Blood count	Leukocytes (10^3 / μL)				
	PN N (10^3 / μL)				
	PN E (10^3 / μL)				
	PN B (10^3 / μL)				
	Monocytes (10^3 / μL)				
	Red blood cells (10^6 / μL)				
	Hemoglobin (g/dL)				
	VGM (fL)				
	Lymphocytes (10^3 / μL)				
	Platelets (10^3 / μL)				
Transaminases	ALAT (UI/L)				
	AST (UI/L)				
Amylase (UI/L)					
Creatininemia (μmol/L)					
Triglycerides (mmol/L)					
Cholesterol level (mmol/L)					
Blood glucose (mmol/L)					
Gender					
Age					
Marital status					

Profession				
Therapeutic compliance				

Collection authorization :

MINISTERE DE LA SANTE ET
DE L'HYGIENE PUBLIQUE
- - - - - - - - - - -
SECRETARIAT GENERAL
- - - - - - - - - - -
CENTRE HOSPITALIER UNIVERSITAIRE
YALGADO OUEDRAOGO
- - - - - - - - - - -
DIRECTION GENERALE
- - - - - - - - - -
DEPARTEMENT DE SANTE PUBLIQUE

2023- - - - - - - -MSHP/SG/CHU-YO/DG/DSP/SPIH

BURKINA FASO
- - - - - - - -
Unité - Progrès Justice

Ouagadougou, le 2 4 FEV 2023

LE DIRECTEUR GENERAL

Au

Pr H. Noëla Estelle YOUL

<u>Objet</u> : Autorisation de collecte de données

J'accuse réception de votre demande relative à l'objet ci-dessus par laquelle vous demandez une autorisation de collecte de données au profit l'étudiant **SOME Sampiouroman** dans le cadre de l'élaboration de sa thèse dont le thème «Etude des paramètres biologiques de tolérance des protocoles antirétroviraux à base du Dolutegravir au Burkina Faso en 2022»

En réponse, j'ai le plaisir de vous informer que je marque mon accord pour le déroulement de ladite collecte.

Cependant l'étudiant SOME Sampiouroman est tenu de bien vouloir déposer une copie finale de sa thèse au département de santé publique.

Pour les modalités pratiques, il voudra bien prendre attache avec le responsable du service concerné.

Tout en vous souhaitant une bonne réception, veuillez recevoir, mes salutations.

<u>**Ampliation**</u> **:**
- Intéressé (e)
- DSP
- Pharmacie

<u>Ousmane NERE</u>
Chevalier de l'Ordre de l'Etalon

RESUME/ABSTRACT

SUMMARY

Title: Study of the biological parameters of tolerance of HIV PL followed under ARV protocols including Dolutegravir in the dermatology and internal medicine departments of the CHU-YO in 2022..

Objective: To describe the biological adverse events of HIV patients on ARV protocols including dolutegravir in 2022 in the CHU-YO.

Materials and methods: This was a retrospective longitudinal study with data collection, the source of which was the patient file of PLHIV followed on DTG between December 2020 and December 2022. The variables considered included blood counts (hemoglobin, leukocyte, lymphocyte and platelet counts), creatinine levels, transaminases (ALAT/ASAT), blood glucose and amylase levels.

Results: A total of 151 Dolutegravir-treated patients with laboratory tests at initiation and after 6 months of treatment were selected and included in the study. The mean age of the patients was 45 years, with extremes of 17 and 89 years. HIV1 infection was the most common type of infection (95.4%), and the TLD protocol was also in the majority (91.4%). The blood count was generally normal. There were no significant changes except in hemoglobin. Indeed, we obtained a decreasing rate of moderate anemia between initiation and 6 months after treatment (41% and 14% respectively). Biochemically, creatinine levels were relatively high after 6 months' treatment compared with initiation, but remained normal (83.48μ mol/L). As for transaminases, we observed an increase in the ASAT level to 45.93IU/L at M6.

Conclusion: Dolutegravir-based protocols are reported to have fewer adverse effects on HIV-positive patients who adhere strictly to treatment regimens. However, it is important to investigate the hepatotoxicity of these ARV protocols including Dolutegravir.

Key words: PV VIH- Biological parameters- Tolerance- ARV- Dolutegravir

Author: Sampiouroman SOME

Email : sampiourosome@gmail.com

Tel: 77233103/73947852

SUMMARY

Title: Study of the biological parameters of tolerance of HIV PV followed under ARV protocols including Dolutegravir in the dermatology and internal medicine departments of the CHU-YO in 2022.

Objective: Describe the biological adverse effects of HIV PV on ARV protocol including Dolutegravir in 2022 in the CHU-YO.

Materials and methods: This was a retrospective longitudinal study with data collection, the source of which was the patient file of PLHIV followed on DTG between December 2020 and December 2022. The variables considered were, among others, blood count (blood count rate). hemoglobin, leukocytes, lymphocytes and platelets); serum creatinine, transaminases (ALT/ASAT), blood sugar, amylase.

Results: In total, 151 patient files on Dolutegravir with biological assessments at initiation and then after 6 months of treatment were retained and included in the study. The average age of the patients found was 45 years with extremes of 17 and 89 years. HIV1 infection was the most represented 95.4% and the TLD protocol was also the majority 91.4%. The blood count was generally normal. There was no significant change except in the case of hemoglobin. Indeed, we obtained a decreasing moderate anemia rate between initiation and 6 months after treatment (41% and 14% respectively). Biochemically, serum creatinine had a relatively high level after 6 months of treatment compared to initiation but still remained normal (83.48 mol/L). As for transaminases, we observed an increase in the AST level to 45.93UI/L at M6.

Conclusion: Protocols based on Dolutegravir would have fewer adverse effects on HIV-positive people who strictly adhere to treatment.

However, it is important to investigate the hepatotoxicity of these ARV protocols including Dolutegravir.

Keywords: HIV PV- Biological parameters- Tolerance- ARV- Dolutegravir

Author: Sampiouroman SOME

Email : sampiourosome@gmail.com

Phone number: 77233103/73947852

GALEN'S OATH

E GALIEN'S OATH

"I swear in the presence of the masters of the faculty, the advisors of the Order of Pharmacists and my fellow students:

To honor those who have instructed me in the precepts of my art and to show my gratitude by remaining faithful to their teaching;

To exercise, in the interest of public health, my profession with conscience and to respect not only the legislation in force, but also the rules of honor, probity and disinterestedness;

Never to forget my responsibility and duty towards the patient and his human dignity.

Under no circumstances will I agree to use my knowledge and status to corrupt morals and promote criminal acts.

May men esteem me if I am faithful to my promises.

May I be covered with opprobrium and despised by my colleagues if I fail to do so".

MINISTERE DE L'ENSEIGNEMENT SUPERIEUR,
DE LA RECHERCHE ET DE L'INNOVATION
****

UNIVERSITE JOSEPH KI ZERBO

****

UNITE DE FORMATION ET DE RECHERCHE
EN SCIENCES DE SANTE (UFR/SDS)

****

SECTION PHARMACIE

****

03 BP : 7021 OUAGADOUGOU 03
TEL : 25-33-73-97 FAX : 25-33-73-98

BURKINA FASO
Unité – Progrès - justice

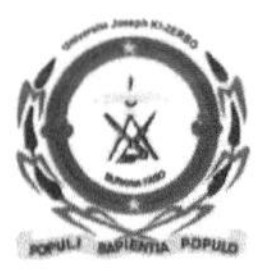

Ouagadougou, 02 Mai 2024

ATTESTATION DE CORRECTION

Nous soussignons **Professeur Éstelle N.H. YOUL** (Professeur titulaire en Pharmacolgie) Directrice de thèse et **Professeur Elie KABRE** (Professeur titulaire en Biochimie) Président du Jury, certifions que le **Docteur SOME Sampiouroman** a apporté les corrections à la thèse intitulée : « **EVOLULION DES PARAMETRES BIOLOGIQUES DE TOLERANCE DES PV VIH SUIVIES SOUS PROTOCOLES ARV INCLUANT LE DOLUTEGRAVIR DANS LES SERVICES DE DERMATOLOGIE ET DE MEDECINE INTERNE DU CHU-YO EN 2022** », conformément aux recommandations des membres du jury le jour de sa soutenance (18/04/2024) de Doctorat en pharmacie (diplôme d'Etat).

Directrice de thèse

Pr Estelle N. H. YOUL

Président du jury

Pr Elie KABRE

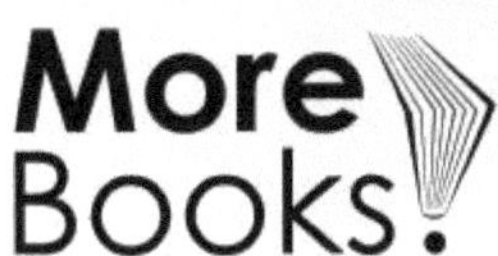
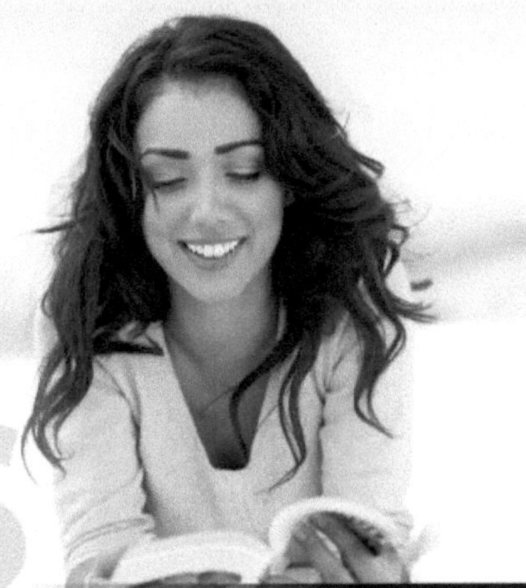

I want morebooks!

Buy your books fast and straightforward online - at one of world's fastest growing online book stores! Environmentally sound due to Print-on-Demand technologies.

Buy your books online at
www.morebooks.shop

Kaufen Sie Ihre Bücher schnell und unkompliziert online – auf einer der am schnellsten wachsenden Buchhandelsplattformen weltweit! Dank Print-On-Demand umwelt- und ressourcenschonend produziert.

Bücher schneller online kaufen
www.morebooks.shop

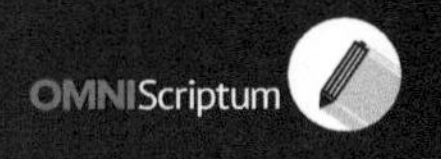

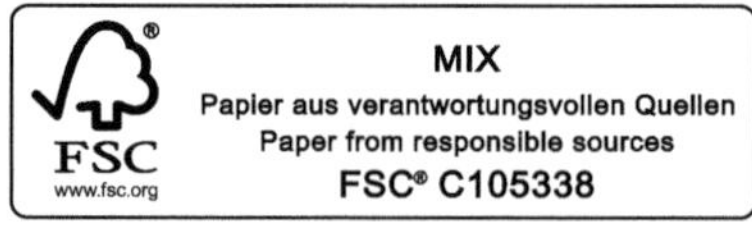

Printed by Books on Demand GmbH, Norderstedt / Germany